M000024226

Awesome Self-Care Face Masks

How to Make the Homemade Face Masks That Keep Your Skin Invigorated and Glowing

BY

Jenny Kings

Copyright 2019 Jenny Kings

License Notes

No part of this Book can be reproduced in any form or by any means including print, electronic, scanning or photocopying unless prior permission is granted by the author.

All ideas, suggestions and guidelines mentioned here are written for informative purposes. While the author has taken every possible step to ensure accuracy, all readers are advised to follow information at their own risk. The author cannot be held responsible for personal and/or commercial damages in case of misinterpreting and misunderstanding any part of this Book

Table of Contents

Homemade Face Mask Recipes

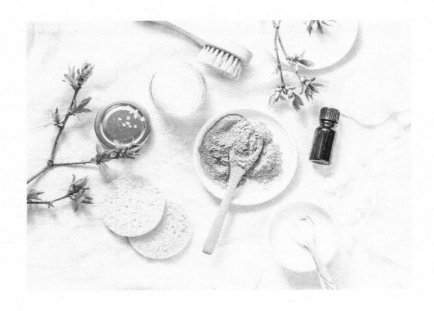

oooooooooooooooooooooooooooooooooooo

(1) Super Green Facial Mask

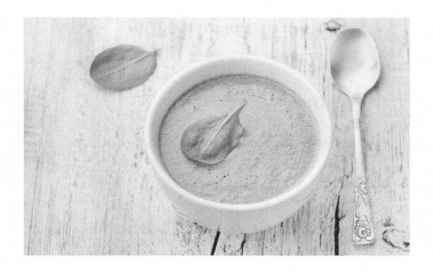

Leafy greens are definitely a healthy choice when it comes to including vitamins and minerals in your diet, so you can imagine how good for your skin this mixture would be. The vitamin C in spinach helps with skin elasticity and you will feel refreshed after you remove the mask. You will feel your skin is much smoother and the radiance of your skin will definitely be noticeable.

List of Ingredients:

- 1/3 cup baby spinach leaves
- 1 tablespoon almond oil
- 2 tablespoons lime juice

Total Prep Time: 20 minutes

OOOOOOOOOOOOOOOOOOOOOOOOOOOOOOOOOOOOOO

Procedure:

Chop the spinach leaves as small as possible; if you want to use the food processor, you can do so but make sure it does not become too watery.

Add the almond oil and lime juice, mix well.

You will look like an alien for sure when you apply the mask all over your face, but you will enjoy the benefits!

Leave it on for 15 minutes.

Always rinse off carefully with warm water and a clean washcloth until the entire facial mask is gone.

(2) Relaxing Apple Facial Mask

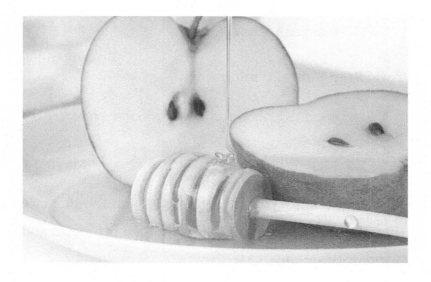

The apple is a very popular fruit and for good reason. It can now be even more popular by using it on your skin. The vitamin C it contains helps you boost your production of collagen which is directly related to your skin's health and elasticity. The vitamin A in apples help decrease the risks of skin cancer, which is awesome! Finally, the copper offered in apples will protect you against ultraviolet rays.

List of Ingredients:

- 1 medium Red Delicious apple (peeled, cored and chopped)
- 2 tablespoons maple syrup
- ½ teaspoons lime juice

Total Prep Time: 20 minutes

oooooooooooooooooooooooooooooooooo

Procedure:

To get the texture you are looking for, you should place the apple and other ingredients in a food processor and blend until smooth.

Apply the mixture all over your dry face. Let it sit for 10-12 minutes.

Always rinse off carefully with warm water and a clean washcloth until the entire facial mask is gone.

(3) Green Tea Homemade Mask

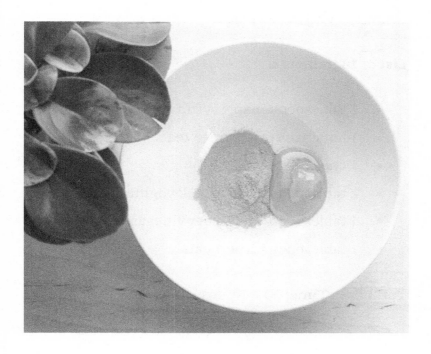

I drink green tea, hot or cold, quite frequently. Now, it's time to also use it as a facial mask. Green tea will help flush out the toxins in your body. The tea's properties can also improve the complexion and the elasticity of your skin. Similarly, it may be able to significantly reduce inflammation because it contains a large amount of antioxidants. Actually, a little additional tip is to use cooled, infused green tea bags directly on your closed eyes to reduce dark circles and puffiness. Leave the tea bags on for about 30 minutes or use the mixture below for a full facial mask.

List of Ingredients:

- 1 tablespoon maple syrup
- 1 pouch of strong green tea
- 1 cup boiling water
- 2 tablespoons plain Greek yoghurt
- 1 tablespoon apple cider vinegar
- 1 tablespoon instant oats

Total Prep Time: 20 minutes

OOOOOOOOOOOOOOOOOOOOOOOOOOOOOOOOOOOOOO

Procedure:

Prepare the green tea as you normally would and then add the instant oats and mix well in a bowl or cup.

Add the rest of the ingredients and mix again. Let it cool completely.

Apply to your face and rest with closed eyes for 20 minutes.

Always rinse off carefully with warm water and a clean washcloth until the entire facial mask is gone.

(4) Smooth Avocado Facial Mask

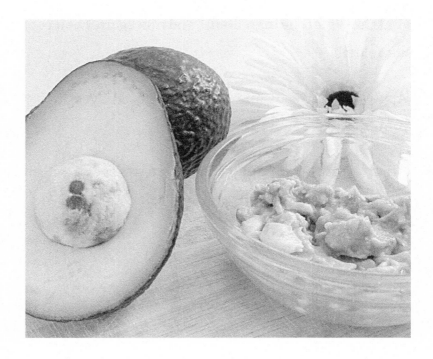

Avocado is definitely a delicious fruit and so smooth! You can imagine how good it will feel when you apply it on your face. Apparently, avocados are awesome at reducing the formation of wrinkles, helping you to fight signs of aging. It can also treat certain skin conditions related to inflammation. The concentration of antioxidants in the fruit will help detoxify your body and your skin, leaving your skin smooth and healthy as can be.

List of Ingredients:

- ½ a ripe medium size avocado (peeled)
- 2 tablespoons agave syrup
- ½ teaspoons coconut oil

Total Prep Time: 20 minutes

OOOOOOOOOOOOOOOOOOOOOOOOOOOOOOOOOOO

Procedure:

Make sure your avocado is very ripe and sliced thinly.

Place the avocado in a bowl with the coconut oil and mash the two together with a fork. Add the agave syrup and mix.

You don't want to use a blender since you don't want the mask to be slushy, but creamy.

Apply on your face avoiding your eyes, of course.

Leave it on for about 15 minutes.

Always rinse off carefully with warm water and a clean washcloth until the entire facial mask is gone.

(5) Two Different Blueberry Facial Mask Ideas

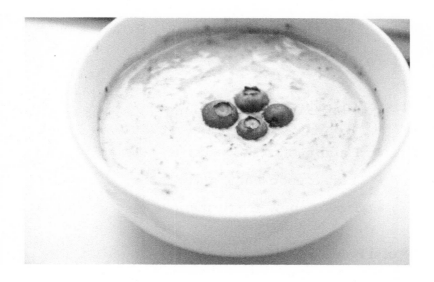

Blueberries are considered one of the richest fruits in antioxidants and prevent many diseases when ingested (including memory loss), and can help slow down the aging process. So, it's not surprising that they are super aids when it comes to bettering your skin. One component in blueberries that we sometimes forget is the level of vitamin C it offers, and this helps blood vessels repair any "broken" or "spider" veins you might see on your face or any other part of your body.

Overall, when using blueberries in your facial mask recipes, you will help your skin stay bright, young, and natural- looking as long as possible. This is one of the most efficient homemade facial mask recipes out there, believe me.

Idea #1

List of Ingredients:

- Handful of fresh blueberries
- 1 tablespoon lemon juice
- Pinch of powered turmeric

Total Prep Time: 20 minutes

OOOOOOOOOOOOOOOOOOOOOOOOOOOOOOOOOOOOO

Procedure:

Mash the blueberries and other ingredients in a bowl.

Apply all over your face and neck (I do front and back).

Leave on for about 15 minutes.

Always rinse off carefully with warm water and a clean washcloth until the entire facial mask is gone.

Idea 2

List of Ingredients:

- Handful of fresh blueberries
- 1 teaspoon cornstarch
- 1 tablespoon raw honey
- 1 tablespoon rosewater

Total Prep Time: 20 minutes

ooooooooooooooooooooooooooooooooooooo

Procedure:

Mash the blueberries with a fork in a bowl, add the other ingredients and combine well.

Brush evenly all over your face and your neck, if desired.

Let it sit and absorb for about 20 minutes before washing.

Always rinse off carefully with warm water and a clean washcloth until the entire facial mask is gone.

(6) Wonderful Oatmeal Face Mask

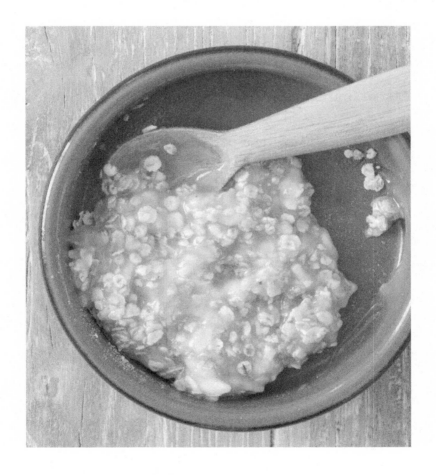

Oats are truly awesome for you and your skin, so why not add them to your facial masks? It actually is a wonderful way to help treat acne and keep your skin moisturized. The oats form a protective layer on your skin and it can cure some minor symptoms such as dryness, rashes, or even itchiness. If you have an unexpected break out, apply this mask we are suggesting and you will be amazed at the results.

List of Ingredients:

- 1/3 cup instant oatmeal (no added sugars or flavorings)
- ½ cup hot purified or spring water
- 1 tablespoon maple syrup
- 2 tablespoons unsweetened plain Greek yoghurt

Total Prep Time: 20 minutes

OOOOOOOOOOOOOOOOOOOOOOOOOOOOOOOOOOOOOO

Procedure:

Combine the oats and hot water in a bowl and stir as if you were making oatmeal.

Add the yoghurt and the maple syrup and stir again.

Apply all over your face avoiding eyes, leaving on for 10-12 minutes.

Always rinse off carefully with warm water and a clean washcloth until the entire facial mask is gone.

(7) A Pumpkin-Based Facial Mask

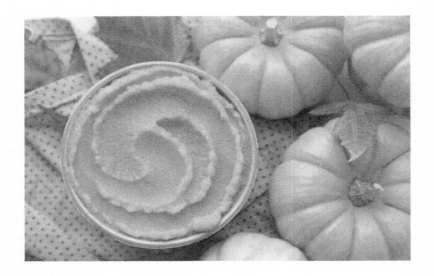

In fall you often have more pumpkins than you can handle! Don't worry, we have a fabulous idea on how to use your leftover pumpkins: make this incredibly refreshing and healthy facial mask. It could be a family activity, too, because usually around Halloween people get together to carve pumpkins, so organize a second party where the girls (and boys, if they want to) can create their own homemade mask. Pumpkins are full of goodness, including the following: antioxidants, vitamin A, vitamin C and enzymes. These components help you keep your skin clear, bright, and smooth. Also, vitamin C is known to help boost collagen production and this means that your skin will receive the benefit of excellent elasticity. We can assure you that you will enjoy preparing and smelling this mask!

List of Ingredients:

- 2 cups of fresh cooked pumpkin flesh or pumpkin puree (unsweetened or even better, organic) from a can
- 3 tablespoons sour cream
- 2 tablespoons honey or maple syrup

Pinch of cinnamon

Total Prep Time: 20 minutes

OOOOOOOOOOOOOOOOOOOOOOOOOOOOOOOOOOOO

Procedure:

If you are using fresh pumpkin flesh, use a blender on low speed to mix it very well with other ingredients so it becomes as smooth as desired.

Apply the final mixture on your face and leave on for 15 minutes.

Always rinse off carefully with warm water and a clean washcloth until the entire facial mask is gone.

(8) The Best Honey Facial Mask Around

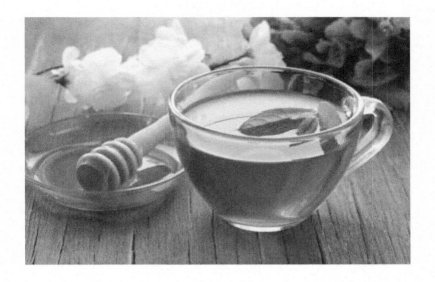

Honey seems such like an obvious choice when it comes to facial masks, but why is that? It smells good and it is natural, yes. But it also has some fantastic properties. Honey is an anti-bacterial so it will clean your pores, help them to breathe, and keep them nice and healthy. It can also fade away some scars or even cases of acne. So, go ahead and add this sweetener to your face mask with no worries.

List of Ingredients:

- 2 chamomile tea bags
- 1 cup hot water
- 1 tablespoon raw honey

Total Prep Time: 20 minutes

ooooooooooooooooooooooooooooooooooooo

Procedure:

Prepare the tea first by boiling the water and infusing 2 bags of tea with 1 cup of water. It will be a concentrated tea mixture.

Let the tea cool down completely before you mix in the honey.

You should have a pasty mix you can apply on your face. Let it sit for about 15-20 minutes.

Always rinse off carefully with warm water and a clean washcloth until the entire facial mask is gone.

(9) Exceptional Papaya Face Mask

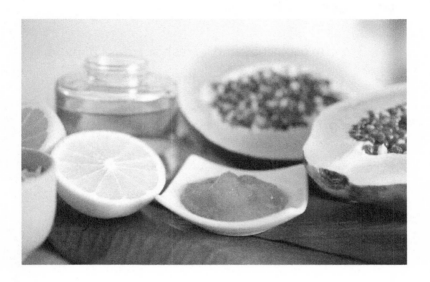

Papaya is not necessarily a fruit you eat every day, I presume. However, it has several advantages including some special skin benefits you might want to look into it. If you read the ingredients on the back of many beauty products, soaps, and shampoos, you will actually discover that papaya is often listed. This beautiful fruit has properties to help your complexion in many ways. For one, it will hydrate your skin, it can remove dead skin cells, and helps slow down the aging process. Finally, it apparently can be quite efficient in lightening skin spots, such as acne blemishes or age spots.

List of Ingredients:

- ½ cup (about ½ fruit) fresh seedless papaya
- 1 tablespoon lemon or lime juice

Total Prep Time: 40 minutes

oooooooooooooooooooooooooooooooooooo

Procedure:

You will need a food processor or blender for this recipe.

Remove all the seeds from the papaya (once you have cut it lengthwise and chopped it in pieces.)

Add all the ingredients in the blender or processor and blend until smooth.

Apply evenly on your face and leave on for about 20 minutes-30 minutes

Always rinse off carefully with warm water and a clean washcloth until the entire facial mask is gone.

(10) Matcha Green Tea Facial Mask

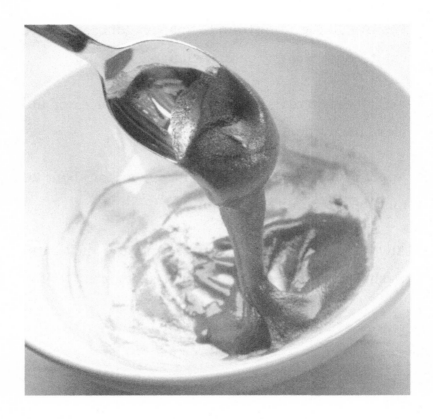

These days, you will find many recipes that include matcha green tea from cookies to breads, sauces, and now facial masks, of course. This powdered mixture offers so many health benefits, we'll tell you about some here. It acts as UV-ray protector, helping your skin from aging too soon, and looking unhealthy. It also gives your skin a boost and detoxifies skin cells, so treat yourself weekly with this facial mask and your skin will definitely thank you.

List of Ingredients:

- 1 tablespoon matcha green
- 1 tablespoon maple syrup or raw honey

Total Prep Time: 20 minutes

ooooooooooooooooooooooooooooooooooooo

Procedure:

In a small bowl, carefully mix the ingredients.

Add a little water if you feel like the consistency is too thick.

Apply all over your face and let it sit for 15-20 minutes.

Always rinse off carefully with warm water and a clean washcloth until the entire facial mask is gone.

(11) No More Puffy Eyes Facial Mask

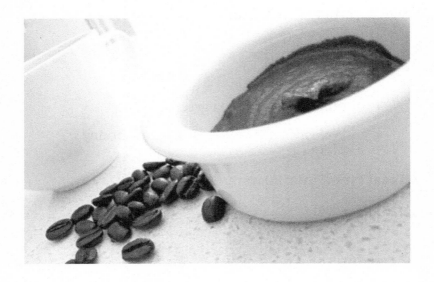

This mask will truly feel like an exfoliator because of the ground coffee texture. You will love the results since coffee offers a few distinctive benefits in skin care. For example, it will help you get rid of dead skin cells. It can also work really well at decreasing puffiness and dark circles under your eyes. Who doesn't want to get rid of those? Coffee offers antioxidants that are responsible for repairing your skin from many types of damage, including too much sun exposure. So now, you can drink your coffee in the morning, and once in a while also apply a ground coffee mask to your face and enjoy the full benefits coffee offers.

List of Ingredients:

- 2 tablespoons of your favorite ground coffee
- 1 Tablespoon honey
- 3 tablespoons light sour cream

Total Prep Time: 20 minutes

OOOOOOOOOOOOOOOOOOOOOOOOOOOOOOOOOOOOOO

Procedure:

Mix all the listed ingredients in a bowl very well.

Proceed to apply all over your face and relax for 15-20 minutes.

Always rinse off carefully with warm water and a clean washcloth until the entire facial mask is gone.

(12) A Pomegranate Facial Mask for Everyone

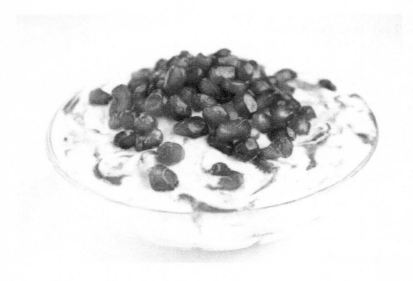

I can't say that I eat pomegranates very often, just because I don't always find them at the grocery store, and honestly don't think about buying them. But once I learned there are many skin health benefits associated with this fruit I made it a point to pick up a few once a month or so and whip up the following recipe. The seeds contain a lot of antioxidants and vitamin C, both components that can help slow down the aging process. So, let's get ready to feel and look younger, shall we?

List of Ingredients:

- 2 tablespoons pomegranate seeds
- ½ cup rolled oats
- 1 tablespoon agave syrup
- 2 tablespoons sour cream

Total Prep Time: 20 minutes

оооооооооооооооооооооооооооооооооо

Procedure:

First of all, place the seeds in a food processor and reduce to a powder.

Place the mixture into a bowl and add the agave syrup and rolled oats, combining well.

Apply all over your face; right away you will feel the exfoliation. Leave on for 10 minutes or so.

Always rinse off carefully with warm water and a clean washcloth until the entire facial mask is gone.

(13) Anti-Aging Mask Made with Grapeseed Oil

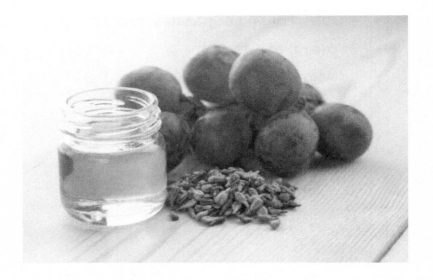

Many types of oils are great to use on your skin for different reasons, but why is grapeseed oil awesome for you? First of all, check out some of your favorite skin products and you might be surprised to find grapeseed oil in the ingredient list. Apparently, grapeseed oil will help scars heal up fast and will also delay wrinkles. The components called polyphenols in this oil act as an anti-inflammatory and will surely help slow down the aging process. Good stuff all around, so don't wait any longer to try it.

List of Ingredients:

- 2 tablespoons grapeseed oil
- 1 tablespoon instant oats or almond flour
- ¼ cup apple cider vinegar
- 1 tablespoon chia seeds

Total Prep Time: 20 minutes

ooooooooooooooooooooooooooooooooooooo

Procedure:

In a mixing bowl combine all ingredients. Let the mixture rest for about 15-20 minutes at room temperature, because the chia seeds and oatmeal will expand.

Apply all over your neck and face and let it sit for at least 10-15 minutes.

Always rinse off carefully with warm water and a clean washcloth until the entire facial mask is gone.

(14) Cider Vinegar Unique Facial Mask

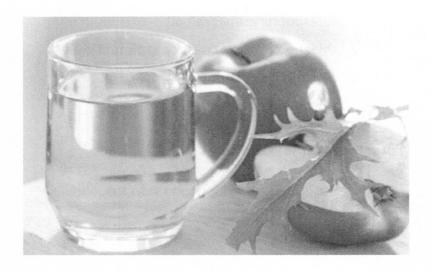

I've heard so many times how good apple cider vinegar is for me and that I should actually drink it, as it will cleanse my body. Today I will indicate how to concoct an effective facial mask. I love how this vinegar leaves my skin fresh and clean, but also how truly competent it can be at reducing age spots, pimples, and wrinkles, because it can help balance the oils on your skin and that is always a good thing. Do not apply only vinegar directly on your skin, it can be too acidic and irritate your skin.

List of Ingredients:

- 1 tablespoon apple cider vinegar
- 1½ cup hot water

Total Prep Time: 20 minutes

OOOOOOOOOOOOOOOOOOOOOOOOOOOOOOOOOOOOOO

Procedure:

Heat the water and mix the vinegar in.

Make sure it is well combined and cooled before applying.

Let it dry on your face.

Always rinse off carefully with warm water and a clean washcloth until the entire facial mask is gone.

(15) Strawberries and Lemon Exfoliating Mask

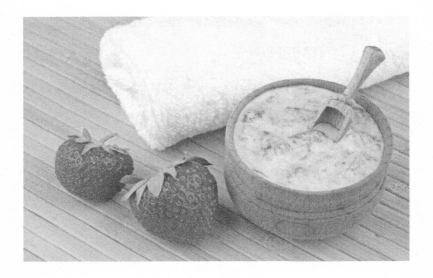

Strawberries are definitely one of my favorite fruits to eat, and now they're one of my favorite ingredients to add to my homemade face masks as well! Because these berries contain salicylic acid, they are actually great at treating or preventing acne, so let your teenagers use the mask once in a while, too. Adding lemon juice to the concoction will remove dead skin cells. Vitamin C-rich strawberries also play a role in helping your pores to breathe better, in reducing oily skin and in fighting signs of aging.

List of Ingredients:

- ¼ cup fresh sliced strawberries
- 1 tablespoon lemon juice
- 1 tablespoon lime juice
- 1 tablespoon honey
- 1 tablespoon sour cream

Total Prep Time: 20 minutes

OOOOOOOOOOOOOOOOOOOOOOOOOOOOOOOOOOOOO

Procedure:

Use a fork to mash all ingredients together in a mixing bowl.

Apply all over your face and let sit for about 10 minutes.

Always rinse off carefully with warm water and a clean washcloth until the entire facial mask is gone.

(16) One of The Most Famous Cucumber Facial Masks

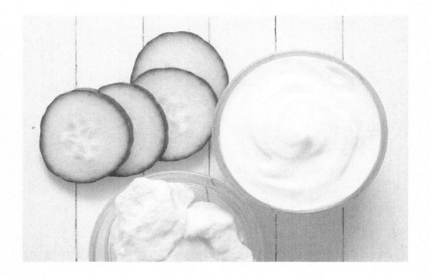

I'm sure you've seen people lying back with some cucumbers slices covering their eyes before! You can do so too, or you can create this special facial mask I suggest below. It's amazing how much of a cooling effect the cucumbers have and I'm always so excited to try one. This mixture is especially good for cooling down your skin, so if you get sunburned, for example, this is the best mixture to apply to your skin. It does not have to be applied only on your face; you can apply it anywhere you'd like.

List of Ingredients:

- ½ small seedless cucumber, peeled
- 1 tablespoon raw honey
- 1 tablespoon Greek plain yoghurt or sour cream

Total Prep Time: 20 minutes

ooooooooooooooooooooooooooooooooooooo

Procedure:

After peeling the cucumber use a fork to mash it well it. Add the honey and yogurt or sour cream. Combine well. (You could also use a food processor, just make sure you don't run it until it's liquid).

Apply all over your face and let it sit for 15 minutes, enjoy!

Always rinse off carefully with warm water and a clean washcloth until the entire facial mask is gone.

(17) Surprising Beer Mask

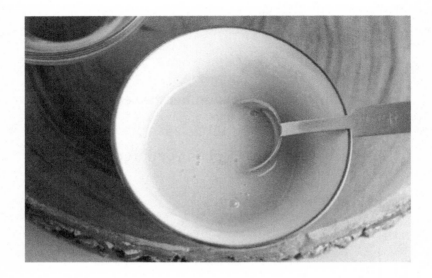

Stop drinking, start applying! That's right, this might be news to you, but beer can actually improve your skin's health quite a bit, so go ahead and use it in your next facial mask recipe. Beer contains starch and barley and this helps your skin get the nourishment it needs. This bubbly beverage will aid you in looking and feeling better by improving your skin's elasticity and decreasing age spots. If you or your loved one is also struggling with acne, have them try the mask; it can help that, too.

List of Ingredients:

- ½ cup beer (any brand works but why not using your favorite kind? Mine is blond)
- ½ teaspoons almond extract
- 1 egg white

Total Prep Time: 20 minutes

ooooooooooooooooooooooooooooooooooooooo

Procedure:

Simply mix all the ingredients together very well and apply on your dry face.

Leave it for about 10 minutes before removing.

Always rinse off carefully with warm water and a clean washcloth until the entire facial mask is gone.

(18) Chai Tea Is an Awesome Mask

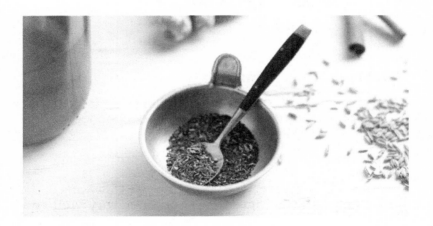

If you would like to improve your skin condition, specifically dryness, puffiness under the eyes, swelling, or even premature aging, then you should try our special chai tea concoction below. Chai tea provides an especially amazing amount of antioxidants and helps your pores open and breathe better. Finally, as with many other teas or natural ingredients, chai tea can definitely help protect you from the damage caused by exposure to UV rays.

List of Ingredients:

- ½ teaspoons chai tea
- 1 cup hot water
- 1 tablespoon maple syrup
- Pinch cinnamon

Total Prep Time: 20 minutes

OOOOOOOOOOOOOOOOOOOOOOOOOOOOOOOOOOOO

Procedure:

Prepare the chai tea with the hot water in a cup or a bowl so you don't have to transfer it later.

Let it cool down and add the maple syrup and cinnamon, combining really well.

Brush all over your face and let it sit about 10 minutes.

Always rinse off carefully with warm water and a clean washcloth until the entire facial mask is gone.

(19) Mask with Spirulina

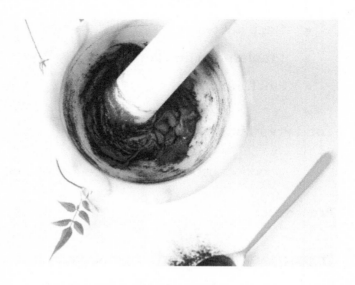

First of all, let's demystify what exactly spirulina is. It is a superfood, no doubt about it, and is sold in powdered form. This powder is blue-green and is rich in nutrients, making it great for your skin as well. It contains beta-carotene, vitamin B-12, and proteins. Apply it on your skin and you will help detoxify and tone it. You will also fight the aging process with this awesome ingredient.

List of Ingredients:

- ½ teaspoons spirulina powder
- ½ mashed avocado
- 1 tablespoon fresh lemon juice

Total Prep Time: 20 minutes

OOOOOOOOOOOOOOOOOOOOOOOOOOOOOOOOOOOOO

Procedure:

Use a fork and mash together the avocado and other ingredients. Make sure the avocado is very ripe.

Apply the mixture on your face and neck and let it sit for 15 minutes.

Always rinse off carefully with warm water and a clean washcloth until the entire facial mask is gone.

(20) Orange Juice Makes Wonderful Facial Masks

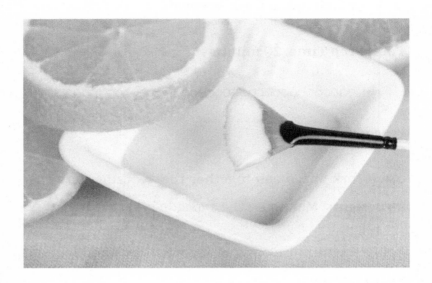

What can be more refreshing than a facial mask made with orange juice? Let us explain why it is so beneficial for your skin as well: Oranges contain vitamin C, and vitamin C is one of the best sources of antioxidants you can give your body and skin; it helps your skin become clearer, cleaner, and removes dead skin cells. Also, the vitamin B in oranges can seriously improve the blood flow in skin, helping with your overall skin tone.

List of Ingredients:

- 2 tablespoons orange juice
- 1 tablespoon lemon juice
- 1/3 cup raw honey

Total Prep Time: 20 minutes

OOOOOOOOOOOOOOOOOOOOOOOOOOOOOOOOOOOOO

Procedure:

Combine all ingredients in a bowl and apply to your face.

You can leave it up to 30 minutes before removing, so relax.

Always rinse off carefully with warm water and a clean washcloth until the entire facial mask is gone.

(21) Maple Syrup and Oats Facial Mask

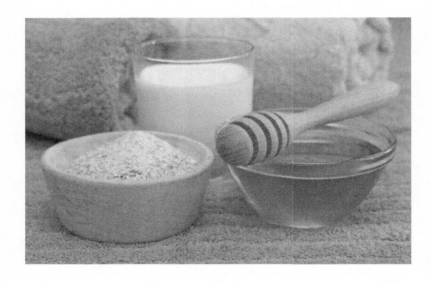

Maple syrup is yummy on pancakes but it's also good for spreading on your skin. Just like honey, maple syrup is great for reducing skin inflammation and dryness. Combined with milk, maple syrup will do wonders for your skin: reduce redness, spots, or any irritation, so apply away! Maple syrup also contains a large amount antioxidants. When mixed with oats, your maple syrup facial mask will give you a wonderful, hydrating effect along with antibacterial properties, keeping your skin extra healthy. Also, just as honey helps you in this area, maple syrup can reduce inflammation or redness of the skin.

List of Ingredients:

- 1 tablespoon warm coconut milk
- 1 tablespoon pure maple syrup
- 1 tablespoon rolled oats

Total Prep Time: 20 minutes

OOOOOOOOOOOOOOOOOOOOOOOOOOOOOOOOOOOOO

Procedure:

Make sure you use pure maple syrup for the recipe and not some imitation kind with preservatives and additives.

Warm up the coconut milk first and then add the maple syrup and the oats, mixing well.

Make sure it is smooth and apply all over your face and neck. Leave it on for 10-15 minutes.

Always rinse off carefully with warm water and a clean washcloth until the entire facial mask is gone.

(22) Spectacular Olive Oil Mask

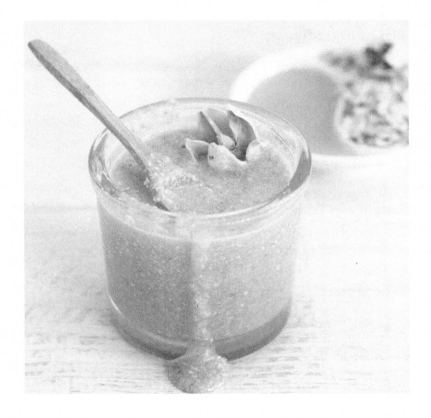

Olive oil is great in the kitchen to cook your food, but did you know it's also wonderful to apply on your skin to help with skin issues and contribute to its health? When combined with an egg yolk, it makes a great consistency to apply on your face. Olive oil is a natural antioxidant so your face will get cleaner and healthier, it will also act as a natural moisturizer and help you kill bacteria on your skin.

List of Ingredients:

- 1 tablespoon agave syrup
- 2 tablespoons olive oil
- ¼ cup rolled instant oats
- 1 egg yolk

Total Prep Time: 20 minutes

oooooooooooooooooooooooooooooooooooooo

Procedure:

Combine all the ingredients.

Apply on your face evenly and let your skin enjoy the benefits for about 15 minutes.

Always rinse off carefully with warm water and a clean washcloth until the entire facial mask is gone.

(23) Simple Brown Sugar Mask

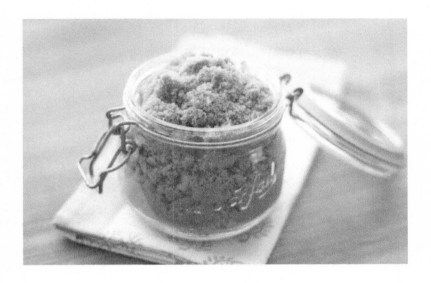

I love the smell of brown sugar when cooking or when I'm applying it to my skin. This natural anti-aging substance will help exfoliate your skin and remove dead skin cells, helping you to glow. You can use this treatment up to twice a week if desired. You can use olive oil instead if desired, I just prefer the smell of the coconut oil myself. I especially love the fresh feeling I get after using this mask. I have been impressed with how well this facial mask can eliminate whiteheads, blackheads, and unclog pores.

List of Ingredients:

- ½ cup brown sugar
- 3 tablespoons coconut oil

Total Prep Time: 20 minutes

OOOOOOOOOOOOOOOOOOOOOOOOOOOOOOOOOOOOOOO

Procedure:

The first step is to reduce the brown sugar into a fine powder: place the brown sugar in a food processor and blend until it's very fine.

In a bowl add the coconut oil to the brown sugar and mix well.

Apply the mask with a circular motion all over your face.

Always rinse off carefully with warm water and a clean washcloth until the entire facial mask is gone.

(24) Very Healthy Organic Banana Mask

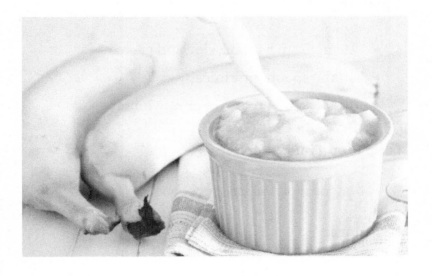

Organic bananas will be a better choice than regular ones because no pesticides are used to grow them. You will benefit from the banana's properties in many ways: to treat acne, help clear age spots, and control your skin's oil levels. Although we are proposing that you peel the banana and mix it with other ingredients, remember that you can always use the banana peel itself. You could apply the inside of the banana peel directly on your skin, especially if you suffer from acne or have visible inflammation, to help soothe it. Potassium in the banana will definitely help moisturize your skin, so help yourself.

List of Ingredients:

- ½ medium banana, ripe and peeled
- 1 tablespoon lime juice
- 1 tablespoon manuka or raw honey

Total Prep Time: 20 minutes

OOOOOOOOOOOOOOOOOOOOOOOOOOOOOOOOOOOO

Procedure:

Mash the half banana in a bowl.

Add the lime juice and the honey and mix all together.

Apply the mixture and leave for 10 minutes.

Always rinse off carefully with warm water and a clean washcloth until the entire facial mask is gone.

(25) Impressive Green Olive Mask

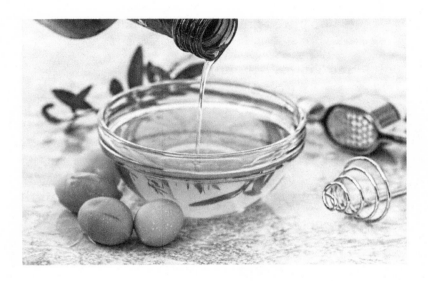

We've already established that olive oil is great for your skin. If you want to go an extra step and use fresh green olives to prepare your facial mask, you can. The vitamin E it contains is a powerful antioxidant that helps your skin looks shinier and cleaner. Also, it can improve the appearance of wrinkles significantly. If you are not crazy about the smell of the natural olive blend, you can add a little brown sugar or honey to the mixture so it's more acceptable. I personally love the smell of olives, so it's never a problem for me.

List of Ingredients:

- ½ cup pitted green olives with natural oils

Total Prep Time: 20 minutes

OOOOOOOOOOOOOOOOOOOOOOOOOOOOOOOOOOOO

Procedure:

Place all the olives in a food processor and blend until it's very smooth.

Apply and leave it on for 15 minutes.

Always rinse off carefully with warm water and a clean washcloth until the entire facial mask is gone.

(26) Cranberry-Filled Facial Mask

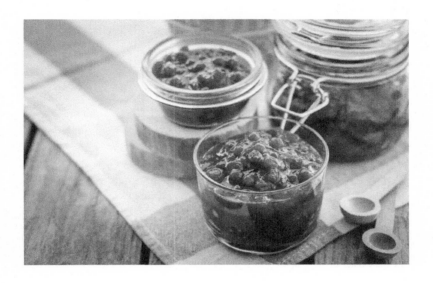

You know cranberries are widely used at Thanksgiving dinner, but let's use them to make a facial mask, as well! Cranberries will provide you with a high level of antioxidants that protect your skin. By applying masks made with cranberries, you can add that layer of protection against aging and UV rays, as well as defending your skin against many infections. Remember, you can always drink cranberries juice to prevent or treat urinary infections, so when applied on your skin you can prevent other types of infection as well. Cranberries will help your skin to keep its balance oil-wise, and can be very useful in treating acne.

List of Ingredients:

- 1 ½ cup fresh cranberries
- 1 tablespoon lemon juice
- 1 tablespoon orange juice
- 1 envelope of unflavored gelatin

Total Prep Time: 20 minutes

OOOOOOOOOOOOOOOOOOOOOOOOOOOOOOOOOOOOOO

Procedure:

You should definitely use an electric mixer or a blender to prepare this mixture. Either way, be careful not to overdo it, you don't want the mixture to become slushy, only creamy.

Apply on your face and enjoy for about 20 minutes.

Always rinse off carefully with warm water and a clean washcloth until the entire facial mask is gone.

(27) Special Greek Plain Yogurt Face Mask

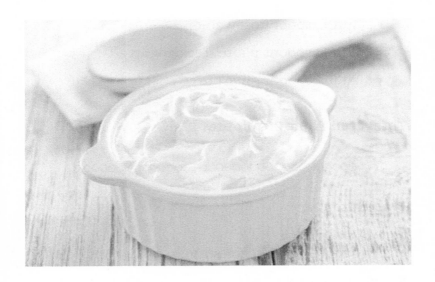

Greek yogurt is certainly getting more and more popular; especially to add on fresh fruit. As far as preparing a nice facial mask, here is how and why you should do it: Yogurt is full of calcium and vitamin D as well as probiotics that will help dissolve dead skin cells. It can also act as a wrinkle and fine line reducer. Most of all, I think you will appreciate how smooth your skin becomes when you apply this mask frequently. You can keep your skin well-hydrated and nicely moisturized with yoghurt.

List of Ingredients:

- 1 tablespoon rosewater
- 2 tablespoons plain Greek yogurt
- 2 tablespoons olive oil

Total Prep Time: 20 minutes

OOOOOOOOOOOOOOOOOOOOOOOOOOOOOOOOOOOOOO

Procedure:

Mix the ingredients together very well. (You will love the smell and feeling of the rosewater on your face, it is so refreshing and delicate.)

Leave on your face for about 15 minutes.

Always rinse off carefully with warm water and a clean washcloth until the entire facial mask is gone.

Author's Afterthoughts

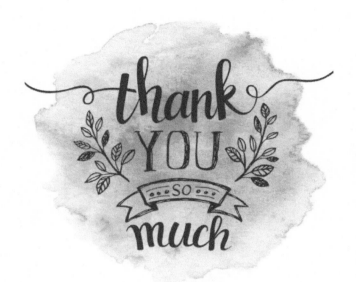

Thank you for reading my book. Your feedback is important to me. It would be greatly appreciated if you could please take a moment to REVIEW this book on Amazon so that we could make our next version better

Thanks!

Jenny Kings

Made in United States
North Haven, CT
20 April 2023